GINKGO BILOBA

The Extraordinary Herb that Boosts Circulation and Enhances Brain Function

Woodland Publishing
Pleasant Grove, UT

© 1996

Woodland Publishing, Inc.
P.O. Box 160
Pleasant Grove, UT 84062

The information contained in this booklet is for educational purposes only and is not recommended as a means of diagnosing or treating an illness. Please consult a professional health care physician knowledgeable in the area of any particular illness or condition. The publisher or author neither directly or indirectly dispense medical advice nor prescribe any remedies, natural or otherwise, and do not assume responsibility for those who choose to treat themselves.

Table of Contents

Ginkgo Biloba   5
   Common Names   5
   Plant Parts   5
   Active Compounds   5
   Pharmacology   5
   Vitamin and Mineral Content   5
   Character   5
   Body Systems Targeted   5

Herbal Forms   5
   Extract   5
   Tincture   6
   Infusion   6
   Capsules   6
   Storage   6
   Regulatory Status   6
   Recommended Usage   6
   Safety   6

History   6

Functions   9
   Increased Brain Power and Memory with Ginkgo   10
   Treating and Preventing Age-Related Mental Disorders   11
   Alzheimer's Disease and Ginkgo   12
   Anti-Stress Herb   13
   Ginkgo: A Natural Antidepressant?   14

Antioxidant Properties of Ginkgo	15
The Cardiovascular System and Free Radicals	15
The Brain's Vulnerability to Oxidants	16
Circulatory System Enhancer	16
A Natural Vasodilator	17
Ginkgo: A Cure for the Common Cold?	18
Smell Perception, Hearing and Ginkgo	18
Ginkgo as a Treatment for Tinnitus	19
Deafness due to Compromised Blood Flow	19
Diabetic Retinopathy and Ginkgo	19
Migraine Headaches and Ginkgo	20
Ginko: A Urinary Tonifier	20
Impotence and Ginkgo	20
Ginkgo: A Hair Tonic that Lowers Cholesterol Levels?	21
The Management of PMS and Ginkgo	21
Ginkgo: An Update	21

Summary of Specific Actions Associated with Ginkgo — 22

Combinations to Enhance Ginkgo — 23

Primary Applications of Ginkgo — 24

Secondary Applications of Ginkgo — 25

Endnotes — 26

Additional References — 28

GINKGO BILOBA
(Ginkgo biloba)

Common Names: maidenhair tree

Plant Parts: leaves

Active Compounds: flavonoid glycosides, diterpenes (including terpene compounds called ginkgolides), bioflavones, quercitin, isorhamnetine kaempferol, proanthocyanidins, sitosterols, lactones, anthocyanin

Pharmacology: The flavoglycosides contained in ginkgo are its most active compounds and have exhibited remarkable pharmacological capabilities. These chemical constituents have free radical properties and function as antioxidants. These flavonoids include quercitin, kaempferol and isorhamnetine. The terpene content of ginkgo, which includes the ginkgolides and the bilobalides help to lessen inflammation by inhibiting PAF (Platelet Activating Factor) in the blood. This action helps to boost circulation. PAF plays a role in diseases such as atherosclerosis, asthma, heart attacks and strokes.

Vitamin and Mineral Content: Ginkgo is rich in bioflavonoids which makes it an effective antioxidant.

Character: astringent, adaptogen, antioxidant, antiseptic, circulatory stimulant, vasodilator and tonic.

Body Systems Targeted: circulatory, cardiovascular, and nervous (brain)

Herbal Forms

Extract: An extract made from ginkgo leaves is available in Europe and is used for cerebral arteriosclerosis in peripheral circulatory disorders of the elderly.

Tincture: Ginkgo tincture is often combined with other herbs such as periwinkle and used for circulatory problems and venous disorders.

Infusion: Infusions of ginkgo are used for arteriosclerosis, varicose veins and hemorrhoids.

Capsules: Powdered forms of ginkgo can be used to enhance brain function and memory.

Storage: Keep in a dark container in a cool, dry environment.

Regulatory Stauts:

U.S.:	none
U.K.:	none
Canada:	none
France:	over-the-counter drug status
Germany:	over-the counter drug status

Recommended Usage: Ginkgo should be taken in normal dosages and, if possible, at the same times every day. In the case of ginkgo, taking it consistently for 12 weeks is recommended. Although injections of Gingko have sometimes been used, oral ingestion of a tablet or capsule is therapeutically effective. More advanced preparations of ginkgo make it possible to obtain higher concentrations of flavoglycosides in smaller amounts of extract.

Safety: Ginkgo extracted from the leaves of the ginkgo tree is considered nontoxic and is virtually without side-effects. It can be safely used with other supplements without interaction and has no reported toxicity. In rare cases, some gastric upset or incidence of headache or skin rash have occurred, which may indicate that the individual is allergic to the substance. The fruit pulp of ginkgo can produce severe contact dermatitis and other allergic reactions. The leaf extract of ginkgo is usually the only form that is available and is extremely safe.

HISTORY

Ginkgo has achieved unprecedented popularity within the last decade and has become a familiar household term. Because interest in treating diseases like Alzheimer's has escalated over the last decade, the biochemical capabilities of ginkgo in regard to brain function have been investigated and are still being researched. Ginkgo is one of those herbs that has become intrinsically connected with notions of herbal elixirs capable of preserving youth and promoting longevity.

Ginkgo comes from the oldest species of tree in the world dating back some 200 million years. Some ginkgo trees have been known to live well over an average of 1000 or more years. The ginkgo tree is also known as the "maidenhair tree" and would have probably become extinct if the trees had not been cultivated in Far Eastern temple gardens and nurtured by Oriental monks.

Ginkgo is a deciduous conifer with separate male and female types. It resembles the pau d'arco tree and like pau d'arco, possesses an unusual immunity to insects and diseases. Ginkgo's remarkable hardiness enabled it to survive the atomic blast at Hiroshima. Because of its unprecedented longevity, ginkgo biloba has sometimes been referred to as a living fossil.

Ginkgo has been used in China for over 5000 years. The Chinese refer to the fruit of the ginkgo tree as *pa-kwo*. This fruit is sold in markets throughout China and resembles dried almonds. Ginkgo fruit is pleasant tasting when fresh, but can become quite disagreeable if allowed to get overly ripe. Asians have relied on extracts of the fan-shaped ginkgo leaf since 3,000 B.C. to heal a wide variety of ailments.

The Chinese have been acquainted with the curative powers of ginkgo for centuries and have typically used the herb for ailments related to aging, such as circulatory disorders, mental confusion and memory loss. In China, ginkgo seeds, called *bai gou,* are considered lung and kidney tonics and are used in conjunction with acupuncture. Ginkgo seeds also help to tonify the urinary system, so they are used in cases of incontinence and excessive urination.[1] Practitioners of Chinese medicine routinely use ginkgo leaves.

Ginkgo was introduced into Europe in 1730 and was well received, not for its medicinal value, but for its ornamental appeal. It is used extensively in landscaping because of its lovely fern-like leaf. It was brought to America in 1784 to the garden of William Hamilton who lived in Pennsylvania.

Decades passed before the healing properties of ginkgo were investigated. Consequently, it has been part of the herbal repertoire only since the 1980s. During this time, it became technically feasible to isolate the essential components of ginkgo. Pharmacologically, there are two groups of substances which are significant compounds found in ginkgo: the flavonoids, which give ginkgo its antioxidant action, and the terpenes, which help to inhibit the formation of blood clots. The majority of scientific interest has focused on Ginkgo's ability to improve the circulation of blood.

Over the past twenty years, scientific testing on the plant has dramatically escalated. Harvard professor Elias J. Corey, Ph.D, synthesized ginkgo's active ingredient, ginkgolide B, for the first time in the laboratory. Consequently, stepped-up research in this country and in Europe resulted. Ginkgo has been the subject of over 300 scientific studies and continues to intrigue scientists. Much modern research has confirmed ancient applications of ginkgo as well as discovered new ones.

Ginkgolide, the active component of the herb, is what creates most of ginkgo's biochemical attributes. Exactly how ginkgolide B functions is not yet known. One theory is that the compound somehow interferes with a chemical found in the body called PAF (platelet activating factor). PAF has been implicated in cases of graft rejection, asthma and other immune disorders. PAF antagonists have been identified from a variety of medicinal plants. These compounds help to explain the pharmacological basis of several traditional medicines and provide a valuable new class of therapeutic agents.

Particular attention has been paid to ginkgo's powerful actions on the cardiovascular system. Thousands of Europeans use this herb for peripheral circulatory disorders. As a circulation booster, ginkgo has accumulated some impressive credentials. Because proper circulation is vital to each and every body function, virtually all body systems can benefit from ginkgo therapy.

Ginkgo's relationship to brain function has also spawned considerable interest. In 1985, Rudolf Weiss said of ginkgo, "Significant improvement in mental states, emotional lability, memory, and the tendency to tire easily, have been reported."

Ginkgo is currently planted in groves and used for a number of medicinal purposes. It is harvested in the summer and can be used in extract, tincture or infusion forms. The therapeutic properties of ginkgo seem endless. Continuing research promises to further uncover additional health benefits of this remarkable botanical. Ginkgo extracts are among the leading prescription medications in France and Germany. Currently, millions of prescriptions for ginkgo are written by physicians worldwide.

FUNCTIONS

Ginkgo may be considered a wonder herb in that it has numerous medicinal applications. Its ability to increase oxygen to living tissue by boosting blood flow makes it invaluable for a number of disorders including heart problems, strokes, and geriatric senility.

Traditionally, the Chinese have used ginkgo to treat bronchial, asthmatic and pulmonary conditions. Recently, research has indicated that certain compounds contained in ginkgo have been shown to effectively dilate arteries, veins and capillaries, which results in increased peripheral blood flow. It is this enhanced circulation of blood which seems to benefit the brain in particular.

Because it effectively boosts brain blood flow, ginkgo may have important potential for treating senility, short-term memory loss, tinnitus (ringing in the ears) and other types of vascular diseases. Ginkgo has been used for Raynaud's disease, intermittent claudication, numbness, vertigo and impotence. It is common practice in Europe and Asia to regularly prescribe ginkgo to improve mental function.

Not commonly known is ginkgo's ability to treat respiratory disorders and stress. It can also function as an excellent antioxidant, due to its bioflavonoid content. Ginkgo also participates in enzyme regulation and protects the blood vessels against plaque build-up and the liver against toxic damage.

Increased Brain Power and Memory with Ginkgo

Ginkgo's ability to enhance cognitive function is becoming common knowledge. Boosting the capability of the brain to record information, communicate ideas or recall concepts can all be enhanced by taking ginkgo biloba therapeutically. Evidently, providing a better oxygen supply to brain cells is ginkgo's primary neural action. The brain is the body's most sensitive organ to oxygen deprivation. Today, more than ever, the effects of smoking, alcohol and stress in general can diminish brain function and compromise mental alertness. Ginkgo has demonstrated over and over that it can make a significant difference in memory retrieval, fact retention and problem solving.

One of the most impressive aspects of ginkgo is its ability to stimulate circulation and oxygen flow to neural tissue, thereby improving cognitive functions and memory. In test cases when ginkgo has been administered, an increase in cerebro-circulation has been noted in both healthy or diseased brain tissue. What makes this finding particularly relevant is that other circulatory enhancers, whether natural or synthetic do not usually possess this capability.

In addition, ginkgo increases oxygen transport at the blood-brain barrier site, while inhibiting the permeability of toxins into brain tissue. As well as boosting blood supply to the brain, ginkgo has demonstrated the ability to increase the rate at which information is transmitted at the nerve cell level.[2]

In a double-blind study, one group of healthy young women received ginkgo extract, and the other was given a placebo. A memory test was administered and the reaction time in those women who had taken the ginkgo improved significantly. These findings corresponded with EEG tracings which showed increased brain wave activity.[3] Short-term memory and basic learning rates can be statistically improved by using ginkgo.

Ginkgo's ability to enhance memory may also be helpful for epileptics who take anticonvulsants. Typically, an anticonvulsant can impair memory function, making it difficult to retrieve names or numbers from memory banks. In addition, although research is lacking, because ginkgo stimulates brain function, it may help to inhibit improper discharging of electrical impulses which is the primary cause of seizures in epileptics.

Ginkgo is rapidly gaining an impressive reputation as a brain enhancer. It has demonstrated its capability to improve memory, mental efficiency and the ability to concentrate. It has also been shown to reduce anxiety, headaches, tension, vertigo, and age-related cerebral disorders. Anyone who has suffered a stroke should look into the possible benefits of ginkgo to amplify mental function and clarity.

Considerable research on ginkgo conducted in Europe has confirmed that ginkgo does indeed facilitate better arterial circulation as well as improve electrical transmission in the nerves. The latter function also contributes to improved oxygenation and nutrition to the brain.[4] Ginkgo is now accepted as a brain booster which improves memory, mental efficiency, cognitive function, communication, orientation and the ability to concentrate. Recently, the notion of using ginkgo for learning disorders has received some attention. Forthcoming research on the subject will help to clarify its potential for treating such conditions.

Treating and Preventing Age-Related Mental Disorders

Ginkgo biloba may be of great value in cases of age-related mental dysfunction including senility, Alzheimer's disease and diminished memory.

In Paris, P. R. Michil conducted a double-blind study in which 50 patients with moderate senile dementia were given either ginkgo or a placebo. Patients treated with ginkgo extract showed a significant improvement in their mood, sociability, and vigilance.

Senility in the elderly is frequently the result of insufficient blood and oxygen flow to brain cells. Anytime this type of insufficiency occurs, short-term memory loss, vertigo, headache, malaise or depression can result. An extract derived from ginkgo leaves offers significant hope to anyone who suffers from diminished blood flow to the brain.

In another large open trial involving 112 geriatric patients who suffered from inadequate cerebral blood flow, 120 mg. of ginkgo biloba extract was administered. The results showed a significant regression of pre-existing symptoms.[5] What this study implies is that so-called "age-related disorders," including senile dementia, may be caused by reduced blood flow to the brain rather than the actual degeneration of nerve cells. Ginkgo appears to increase oxygen utilization in brain tissue, which also enables neural cells to metabolized sugar more effectively.[6]

Alzheimer's Disease and Ginkgo

Concerning Alzheimer's disease, ginkgo has been shown to normalize the acetylcholine receptors in the brain of aged animals which results in an increased transmission of nerve impulses. Alzheimer patients experience a decrease in these very functions.

Clearly, test results have repeatedly shown that ginkgo has a positive effect in geriatric patients who have already experienced a deterioration of their mental performance. For this reason, it should be considered a viable treatment option in cases of Alzheimer's disease and senile dementia. It is important to realize that it appears the ginkgo works more effectively in delaying the mental demise that occurs in the initial stages of Alzheimer's disease. Once the disease is well established, the effects of ginkgo are minimized. On the other hand, if mental deterioration is due to a circulatory insufficiency, ginkgo therapy can help to reverse the condition.

Laboratory tests performed on aged rats showed that ginkgo extract works to protect neuronal membranes in the brain. In addition, these tests also showed that the herb has a restorative effect which can help to prevent the decrease in cerebral receptors that occurs with aging.[7]

Double-blind studies on groups of elderly subjects have confirmed that using ginkgo before presenting tests which required mental processing significantly shortened the time required to process the material, which facilitated a speedier transference of information. Combining ginkgo with panax ginseng had similar results. Tests showed that this combination has a favorable effect on both learning and memory in aged individuals.

Perhaps the most exciting biological potential ginkgo has is the possibility that it may prevent the onset of certain age-related disorders if taken early enough. Research suggests that it may offer significant protection against the development of mental deterioration and strokes. In other words, the diminished mental function which routinely accompanies aging could be significantly prevented with ginkgo therapy.

Anti-Stress Herb

Ginkgo's popularity has steadily increased as more of its properties have been discovered. It has become the subject of widespread interest and was recently the topic of a scientific conference that was held in New York. Because stress management is so crucial to our contemporary lifestyles, the role of ginkgo should not be dismissed. Research has shown that ginkgo can help relieve the adverse effects of stress. It is considered an herbal adaptogen which helps the body cope with a number of physical and psychological stressors.

One way in which ginkgo helps boost stamina is by helping the body conserve energy through the increased biosynthesis of protein and nucleic acids. This process is vital to any kind of healing or cell regeneration. Ginkgo also helps to increase levels of glucose and ATP at the cellular level which helps us sustain higher energy output, especially under periods of mental or physical stress.

Frequently, stress impairs cognitive ability, and because ginkgo facilitates better blood flow to brain neurons, coping abilities may be enhanced.

Several experiments have demonstrated that ginkgo can help to facilitate one's ability to adapt in an adverse environment. Because most of us have to cope with adversity in one form or other, ginkgo may be of benefit in helping to promote better coping skills and enhanced physiological function.

Unquestionably, stress contributes to both physical and emotional disorders. Ginkgo can help protect us against the deleterious effects of stress by making our cellular structures more resilient.

Ginko: A Natural Antidepressant?

Several health practitioners are looking at ginkgo as a possible natural substitute for some pharmaceutical antidepressants. Because ginkgo stimulates the brain through increased oxygen availability, it may have therapeutic value in some cases of depression. Depression is viewed by some doctors as a condition of brain "sleepiness."

By increasing mental alertness, ginkgo may help to snap a depressed brain out of its mental patterns by stimulating biochemical reactions at the cellular level. Ginkgo may inadvertently work the same way that exercise does for people suffering from depression. Exercise helps to oxygenate the blood and by so doing, elevates mood. Ginkgo accomplishes a similar action by boosting brain blood flow. Ginkgo has also been recommended in combination with antidepressant drugs such as tricyclics and tetracyclics. It should be noted that tests using ginkgo to treat depression used higher than normal dosages of ginkgo.

Learning disabilities may also benefit from the neuro-stimulation ginkgo provides, however, no one has studied its effects in this area.

Antioxidant Properties of Ginkgo

Ginkgo also has the capability of decreasing cell damage which results from the presence of free radicals. A free radical is a chemical structure with an unpaired electron. Because of its missing electron, it becomes unstable and randomly impacts other cellular structures causing cellular deterioration. Free radicals can, in a sense, put a chemical hole in body tissues. They are capable of destroying a gene or causing a cell wall to leak fluids. In turn, any cellular damage liberates more free radicals which continues the cycle of on-going cellular damage. Free radicals can alter the behavior of a cell or cause it to mutate or disintegrate. This process can result in degenerative diseases such as cancer, heart disease and premature aging.

Research has shown that ginkgo contains antiradical or antioxidant properties. Myricetin and quercitin are flavonoid constituents contained in ginkgo and are responsible for its scavenging capabilities. Ginkgo extract is known to be efficient in helping to treat or prevent diseases associated with free radicals. The therapeutic action of ginkgo can play a significant role in the treatment of various biological disorders, which are attributed to free radical damage, especially any type of inflammatory condition. Laboratory tests and animal studies have conclusively shown that ginkgo biloba has proven itself to be an extremely effective free radical scavenger.

The Cardiovascular System and Free Radicals

It is the bioflavonoid content of ginkgo which enables the compound to scavenge free radicals so effectively. The flavonoids in ginkgo help protect cells against free radical contact. These flavonoids have an enzyme-regulating effect also found in citru-derived bioflavonoids with one important difference: the efficacy doses reported for ginkgo are much lower. In addition, these bioflavonoids provide protection to blood vessels against the damaging effect of plaque build-up.

Scientists have discovered that is the antioxidant action of ginkgo which helps prevent damage to heart muscle. Ginkgo reduces the formation of free radicals. Ginkgo may provide some protection from exposure to damaging ultraviolet light.

The Brain's Vulnerability to Oxidants

The antioxidant action of ginkgo helps to keep ample supplies of oxygen to brain neurons which are involved in memory retrieval. The flavonoids in ginkgo help to decrease the metabolism of oxidants in brain cells which can help prevent reduced blood flow to brain tissue. The antioxidant properties of ginkgo are most evident in brain tissue, which is made up of nerve cells. Brain cell membranes are compressed of a high percentage of unsaturated fatty acids which make them particularly vulnerable to free radical damage and hypoxia (lack of oxygen).

The brain has little in the way of energy reserves and requires a continual supply of glucose and oxygen. When circulation is compromised, both of these components are reduced. If blood flow is diminished enough, brain cells will die. Ginkgo helps these cells to utilize glucose and boosts oxygen supply. As a result, energy production in brain tissue is enhanced.

Circulatory System Enhancer

An article by Frank Murray in the April 1989 issue of *Better Nutrition* says, "Dr. Huber and Kidd concur with other researchers that ginkgo biloba dilates the blood vessels, allowing greater blood flow to the tissues. It also provides better drainage of waste products, especially through arteries that have been partially blocked because of atherosclerosis."

The article goes on to discuss the fact that ginkgo also inhibits the clumping of blood platelets, which can contribute to heart and artery problems. When circulating platelets stick together on worn areas found on the walls of aging vessels, clots and blockages can form.

Anytime this happens, heart attack and stroke are possibilities. Ginkgolides are unique twenty-carbon terpenes which inhibit PAF (platelet activating factor), which controls the formation of clots.

PAF also plays an important role in other disorders such as asthma, shock, anaphylaxis, renal disease, graft rejection, CNS disorders and a number of inflammatory conditions.

A Natural Vasodilator

Ginkgo affects the lining of the blood vessels and acts to dilate them through a chemical constituent which stimulates the release of a certain factor. Tests have shown that ginkgo extract promotes better venous tone, which helps to clear the blood of toxic metabolites that collect when blood flow is diminished.

Apparently Oriental herbalists used the ginkgo leaf for arterial circulatory problems. Blood vessels can constrict in cases of diabetes, Raynaud's disease, gangrene, angina, and intermittent claudication. Ginkgo can help to relieve leg cramping by facilitating better circulation to the limbs. In addition, it increases the circulation of blood to the retina and can help to prevent macular degeneration.

Concerning heart function, some studies suggest that ginkgo can help normalize heartbeat. Research has shown that ginkolide contained in ginkgo can be as effective as some pharmaceutical drugs in treating severely irregular heartbeats.[8]

Because ginkgo can effectively reduce blood cell clumping, it can help prevent some heart-related disorders such as congestive heart disease. Circulatory impairment is at "the heart" of cardiovascular disease and ginkgo specifically acts to enhance circulation.

Several laboratory tests have found that ginkgo helps the heart contract more effectively after times of stress by reducing the formation of oxygen free radicals. This protective effect can help prevent damage to heart muscle which may become oxygen deprived.

Ginko . . . A Cure for the Common Cold?

In his book, *Secrets of the Chinese Herbalists,* Richard Lucas says, "According to a German newspaper, Dr. Joachim H. Volkner, a nose, ear and throat specialist is Berlin, announced the discovery of a lightning cure for the common cold. Dr. Volkner found that if a person inhales an essence prepared from the leaves of the ginkgo tree, his cold will improve." Two hundred and twenty-four people tried the ginkgo treatment and the results were dramatic, to say the least.

The German report stated, "The inflamed areas healed immediately."[9] Lucas goes on, "Dr. Volkner confesses that he hasn't as yet identified the exact substance in the ginkgo leaves that produces the therapeutic effects, but he does explain how the treatment works. When a person catches a cold, the cells of the mucous membranes are damaged and are unable to store moisture. The efficiency of the cell walls becomes impaired because substances in the cell press against these walls. Apparently, the ginkgo essence forces these components of the cell back into its interior. Dr. Volkner explains that 'the microbes which have collected inside die off, and very shortly after inhalation of the ginkgo essence they completely disappear.'"[10]

Smell Perception, Hearing and Ginkgo

Over 200,000 visits to the doctor annually are due to lack of smell or the diminished ability to smell properly. In addition, an abnormally heightened sense of smell can also be a problem. Interestingly, these types of smell disorders are commonly seen in people suffering from Alzheimer's disease or Parkinson's disease. Both of these disorders are the result of faulty bio-chemical reactions in the brain. Ginkgo is one of the supplements that has been reported to help smell perception. Effective dosages would depend on the degree of severity and the current nutritional status of the person.

Ginkgo as a Treatment for Tinnitus

When circulation is improved, frequently hearing does as well. Ginkgo helps to oxygenate tissues more effectively which can enhance nutrient transport to the nerves of the inner ear. As a result, conditions such as tinnitus (ringing in the ear) may be alleviated. Tinnitus is a very difficult condition to effectively treat. If the tinnitus is the result of a circulatory deficiency, ginkgo may be effective. The role of ginkgo as a viable therapy for the disorder remains somewhat controversial.

In terms of treating tinnitus with ginkgo, experimentation is the best approach. Tinnitus can be caused by a number of different problems and the search for an effective treatment can only be made by the individual. In addition, treatment must be sustained for a long period of time before any judgement can be drawn. A minimum of two weeks is necessary. For more severe cases of tinnitus, a longer period of therapy is required.

German tests using ginkgo for sudden hearing loss suggested that in cases where hearing is lost for no apparent reason, ginkgo was effective in promoting a remission after one week of treatment. In some cases, hearing was also improved.[11] One of the main advantages of using ginkgo over other drugs for hearing loss is that it is considered safe with minimal side effects.

Deafness Due to Compromised Blood Flow

In some cases of cochlear deafness, ginkgo has proven to be a valuable therapeutic agent. As in the case of tinnitus, treatment should be initiated and sustained.

Diabetic Retinopathy and Ginkgo

There is evidence to suggest that ginkgo extract may be beneficial for people with diabetes who risk damage to their optic nerves. Frequently, diabetes causes the membranes of capillaries located in the retina to thicken, thereby obstructing blood flow and reducing vision. The retina is particularly susceptible to free radical damage. Apparently, ginkgo helps protect against that damage by reducing the amount of lipoperoxidation which can cause permanent vision loss.

Laboratory studies using rats found that ginkgo may be able to prevent the impairment of visual function caused by free radicals, which can increase when blood sugar levels are high, and by inhibiting the formation of blood clots in the eye.

Migraine Headaches and Ginkgo

Because ginkgo helps to promote proper cerebral circulation, it may be effective in some cases of migraine headaches. Migraines are believed to be the cause of a malfunction in vasodilation and constriction of blood vessels in the brain. By heightening blood flow and oxygenation of brain tissue, this neuro-vascular disorder may be alleviated or even prevented. More research is required to establish a firm scientific link between migraines and ginkgo.

Ginkgo: A Urinary Tonifier

Ginkgo has been used extensively in China to treat kidney infections, kidney stones and other urinary tract disorders. It is considered valuable because it has a tonifying effect on the urinary system.[12]

Impotence and Ginkgo

Frequently, compromised blood flow to the penis is the primary cause of impotence. In these cases, ginkgo may prove to be very important in treating erectile dysfunctions. Recent tests have indicated that improving the arterial blood flow to penile tissue was accomplished by ginkgo therapy without changing blood pressure. As in the case of hearing loss or tinnitus, the longer the ginkgo was taken the better the results.

Ginkgo: A Hair Tonic that Lowers Cholesterol Levels?

Japanese experiments have recently found that the ethanolic extract found in ginkgo leaves demonstrated the ability to stimulate hair regrowth in mice which had been given a normal and a high butter diet. Test results found that ginkgo extract not only inhibited the increase of serum triglyceride levels in the mice who ate a highly saturated diet, it also significantly promoted the growth of hair in shaved areas.[13] When ginkgo is combined with garlic, a considerable drop in cholesterol levels is also observed. A number of patients with elevated cholesterol levels showed an improvement rate of 35 percent versus a control group.[14] The secret to keeping cholesterol levels consistently low is long-term therapy with garlic and ginkgo. When the extracts were no longer taken, cholesterol levels began to rise again.

The Management of PMS and Ginkgo

Symptoms of PMS usually include water retention, breast tenderness and vascular congestion. One hundred sixty-five women between the ages of 18 and 45 who suffered from significant PMS were tested with ginkgo, which was given from the 16th day of the first cycle to the 5th day of the next. Test studies confirmed that ginkgo was effective against various symptoms of PMS, particularly breast changes. In addition, mental and emotional symptoms associated with PMS also decreased.[15] Because Ginkgo is so safe to use, it may be very beneficial for women who have used drug therapy for PMS that had undesirable side effects.

Ginkgo: An Update

Ginkgo is currently being studied as a safer substitute for anti-rejection drugs which are routinely given to recipients of transplanted organs. Ginkgolide, the active component of ginkgo, somehow inhibits a chemical found in the body called PAF (platelet activating factor) which plays a role in organ rejection. It may also prove beneficial for congestive heart failure, angina, shock, multiple sclerosis and burns.

Summary of Specific Actions Associated with Ginkgo

- Improves blood circulation and oxygenation of brain cells, which boosts brain function and helps to treat disorders such as senile dementia, some types of depression and Alzheimer's disease.
- In stimulating brain cell oxygenation, may significantly improve mental clarity and alertness.
- Strengthens the vascular system, which helps decrease the risk of blood clots, therefore lessening the probability of strokes.
- Tissue oxidation and nutrient transport are enhanced, thereby contributing to the treatment of any vascular disease such as tinnitus in the ear and any macular generation in the eye, as well as leg pain due to arterial insufficiency.
- May contribute to less organ rejection in the case of transplants by inhibiting a compound called PAF (platelet activating factor) which is involved in the rejection process.
- Works as an anti-stress adaptogen herb in its ability to increase ATP at the cellular level, resulting in increased energy and heightened stamina.

Unquestionably, ginkgo will continue to enjoy its current popularity. As baby boomers continue to enlarge the senior citizen block of our population, supplements which have the ability to deter or even prevent age-related disorders will be vigorously sought after.

Ginkgo can be used in these combinations for bioenhancement:

- ginkgo, ginseng, sage, bee pollen, and capsicum
- ginkgo, suma and gotu kola
- ginkgo and garlic
- ginkgo and butcher's broom, centella, milk thistle and bilberry
- ginkgo and vitamin B complex, magnesium, and choline

Ginkgo: Primary Applications

The following are general areas that ginkgo biloba can be used effectively:

- Alzherimer's Disease
- Antioxidant
- Attention Span
- Blood Clots
- Brain Booster
- Cardiovascular Problems
- Cerebrovascular Insufficiency
- Circulatory Disorders
- Dementia
- Dizziness
- Edema
- Hypoxia
- Inflammation
- Impotence
- Ischemia
- Longevity
- Memory Loss
- Multiple Sclerosis
- Muscular Degeneration
- PMS
- Raynaud's Disease
- Senility
- Stress
- Stroke
- Tinnitus
- Vascular Disease

Secondary Applications

The following are areas of secondary application for ginkgo biloba:

- Allergies
- Angina
- Anxiety
- Arthritis
- Asthma
- Bronchial Infections
- Cancer
- Carpal Tunnel Syndrome
- Cough
- Depression
- Epilepsy
- Eye Problems
- Hemorrhoids
- High Blood Pressure
- Lung Conditions
- Migraines
- Toxic Shock Syndrome
- Transplant Rejection
- Urinary Tract Disorders
- Varicose Veins
- Vascular Impotence
- Vertigo

Endnotes

[1] Penelope Ody. *The Complete Medicinal Herbal.* (New York: Dorling-Kindersley, 1993) 64.

[2] I. Hindmarch and Z. Subhan. "The Psychophar-macological Effects of Ginkgo biloba Extract in Normal Healthy Volunteers." *Int. J. Clin. Pharmacol Res.,* (1984), 89-93.

[3] B. Gebner and M. Klasser. "Study of the Long-Term Action of Ginkgo biloba Extract on Vigilance and Mental Performance as Determined by Means of Quantitative Pharmaco-EEG and Psychometric Measurements." *Arzneim-Forsch.* (1985) 35, 1459-65.

[4] James Brady MD. "A Scientific Herb for Symptoms of Aging." *Doctor's Best.* (Laguna Hills, California).

[5] G. Vorberg. "Ginkgo biloba Extract (GBE): A Long-Term Study of Chronic Cerebral Insufficiency in Geriatric Patients." *Clinical Trials Journal.* (1985) 22, 149-57.

[6] Michael Murray N.D., and Joseph Pizzorno, N.D. *Encyclopedia of Natural Medicine.* (Rocklin, California: Prima Publishing, 1991) 34.

[7] F. Juguet, K. Drieu and A. Piriou. "Decreased Cerebral 5-HT1A Receptors During Aging: Reversal by Ginkgo biloba Extract," *J. Pharm. Pharmacol.* 1994 Apr. 46(4): 318-8.

[8] Ody, 64.

[9] *Today's Herbs,* "Ginkgo." (Provo, Utah: Woodland Health Books, September, 1992) 49.

[10] *Today's Herbs,* 50.

[11] F. Hoffmann, C. Beck, A. Schutz and P. Offermann. "Ginkgo Extract EGb 761 (tenobin)/HAES versus naftidrofuryl (Dusodril)/Haes. A Randomized Study of Therapy of Sudden Deafness." *Laryngorhinootologie.* 1994 March 73(3): 149-52.

[12] Rita Elkins. *The Complete Home Health Advisor.* (Pleasant Grove, Utah: Woodland Books, 1994) 233.

[13] N. Kobayashi, R. Suzuki, C. Koide, T. Suzuki, H. Matsuda and

M. Kubo. "Effect of Leaves of Ginkgo biloba on Hair Regrowth in C3H Strain Mice." *Yakugaku-zasshi.* 1993 Oct. 113(10): 718-24.

[14]R. Kaezelmann and F. Kade. "Limitation of the Deterioration of Lipid Parameters by a Standardized Garlic-Ginkgo Combination Product: A Multicenter Placebo-Controlled Double-Blind Study." *Arzneimittelforschung.* 1993 Sept. 43(9): 978-81.

[15]A. Tamborini, and R. Taurelle. "Value of Standardized Ginkgo biloba Extract (EGb 761) in the Management of Congestive Symptoms of Premenstrual Syndrome." *Review Gynecol. Obstet.* 1993 Jul-Sep 88(7-9): 447-57.

Additional References

Auguet, M., V. DeFeudis and F. Clostre. "Effects of ginkgo biloba on arterial smooth muscle responses to vasoactive stimuli." *Gen. Pharm.* 13, 169, 1982.

Bauer, U. "Six month double blind randomized clinical trial of ginkgo biloba extract versus placebo in two parallel groups in patients suffering from peripheral arterial insufficiency." *Arzneimittel Forschung,* 34, 716, 1984.

Peter, H. "Vasoactivity of ginkgo biloba preparation." 4th Conf. Hung. *Ther. Invert. Pharmacol.,* Soc. Pharmacol. Hung. B. Dumbovith, ed., 177, 1968.

Racagni, G. N. Brunello and R. Paoletti. "Neuromediator changes during cerebral aging. The effect of Ginkgo biloba extract." *Presse med.* 15, 310, 1488-90, 1986.